# Weight Los Hacks: 10 SIMPLE and Powerful Hacks That Will Keep YOU Motivated to Lose Weight

*Hack Your Way to Weight Loss!*

Jennifer Cox

# My Story

I really want to thank you for downloading this book and wish you the best of success in implementing these strategies. I wanted to talk about my story – not to be boastful – but to serve as motivation to my readers :)

From a young age my diet consisted of junk food several times a week and anything that I could microwave. I often would hit the drive through 5 times a week. This coupled with little to no exercise meant that I ballooned through my teenage years to eventually **400 pounds**.

It all came one fateful day, when looking at pictures, I couldn't believe what I was seeing. I saw myself as the obese, unhealthy and unattractive woman I was. I went through the infamous cycle of acceptance. At first it was denial, "I'm not THAT big, am I?", "The camera adds 10 (more like 100) pounds" were some of the justifications I used. I eventually slowly began to slide into depression and this lasted several months. I began popping pills to help improve my mood, despite knowing what needed to be done. I eventually reached I stage where I knew I needed to change.

I began exercising, eating right and mixing with the right people. I worked hard and at times it was torture. I began to learn about correct food choices and how bad the food was that I was previously eating. As the pounds started coming off I increased my activity rate and continued with my diet. I was able to bring my weight down to **160 pounds**.

My journey was a long and arduous one, and one which demanded greater mental strength than physical. I have written this book in the hope of motivating people who are also in my position. The focus though is on how to use your mental capacity to reach your goals. The diet plan which you follow is of vital importance, but you won't follow through on it without the acceptance of your mind.

I hope these "hacks" prove helpful to you in reaching your goals, I would love to hear from you on how these have helped you get the body you have always wanted.

# Table of Contents

# Part One: Mind over Matter

"Mind over matter" is an idiom that we often hear in modern speech. But have you really considered what it means? It is the ability to overcome any physical problem through the use of willpower – or your mind. Your mind is one of your greatest treasures and I am now going to teach you how to leverage it and use it to your advantage in achieving your weight loss goals.

## Hack 1: Put Your Mind to It

You must put your mind to losing weight or all the diet plans in the world will not work. The key is to develop a determined mindset which takes precedence over everything else in your life.

When you are at a restaurant and the waitress or waiter asks if you left room for dessert, how do you answer? Do you always say yes and order a dessert? Perhaps due to the cost of restaurant desserts you decline, but then stop somewhere else like the grocery store to get a dessert? If someone offers you pie, cake, or another dessert at a family gathering or special celebration, do you always take the dessert? Most likely you are answering these questions in the affirmative.

How can you change the answer of "yes, I will have dessert" to "no I won't have dessert"? You have to put your mind to it. You have to realize deep within your heart that these foods are going to hinder your overall goal, which is to lose weight.

You have to realize the needlessness of eating junk food, when the overall benefit of eating healthy and losing weight is to feel better physically, emotionally and mentally. Do you want to continue looking in the mirror knowing you are overweight and doing nothing about it? Or, would you like to look in the mirror and say "today I conquered my cravings and ignored the dessert/pizza/pie/pick your poison?"

The best way to conquer junk food and other harmful foods you have eaten in the past is to focus on the reasons why you should not eat them. For example:

1. If you eat dessert or junk food, you may be full or too full.
2. Eating excess foods at meal time will make you feel uncomfortable.
3. Too many carbs will provide short term energy, but leave you feeling tired.
4. The wrong foods can cause fatigue and improper sleep cycles.

These are just a few of the things you can say in your mind to help you get over the hurdle of eating the foods that are bad for you. You are reminding yourself, using your mind, to show you that the "matter" in front of you is not greater than your mindset.

## Hack 2: Know Yourself

Know yourself – hone in on your motivations for weight loss – why are you doing it? What are your strengths and weaknesses? How can these be used to achieve your goals? You have to take a hard look at yourself to answer these questions. You cannot prevaricate the truth about how you perceive your strengths and weaknesses, nor why you are trying to lose weight. If you are not honest at the outset of your new diet and weight loss program, you have the potential to continue failing time and again. Failures are fine, as you will learn later. However, continuing in a cycle of not losing weight, losing confidence, and being unhappy will make it that much harder to be motivated on the next attempt.

The best reason for losing weight is one that is about you. You may want to look great again or you may want to lose weight because of health concerns. Whatever the reason, it should be centered on you and not for foolish reasons. Losing weight because someone calls you names, doesn't find you attractive, or for other people is not going to motivate you enough to stick with the weight loss program you have chosen. Peoples opinion of your body don't matter, it is your opinion of your body that takes precedence.

Right now take out a piece of paper or a journal that you keep. List your reasons for wanting to lose weight, no matter how ridiculous. Then, in another column list your weaknesses and in another your strengths. Are you sure you have each one or that these are accurate weaknesses/strengths? Self-perception can be incorrect due to lack of self-esteem, depression, and other factors. If you find it difficult to see your weaknesses/strengths or accurately assess them, talk it out with someone you trust to tell you the truth. This same person can help you with the strengths column too.

It is best if you come up with them, rather than depending on another, but if you need a little help that is okay. Sometimes a little help allows us to open up to the truth of who we really are. Meditation can be one way to determine your strengths and weaknesses if you are having a little trouble.

Whichever way you determine these, they will provide a blueprint to how you can tackle almost any problem in your life. If we take weight loss as an example, if you know one of your weaknesses is saying "no" to junk food, how about you inform your family/friends/colleagues that you are on a diet to better yourself. In this way they will not tempt you with bad foods. If you get easily demotivated, how about finding a buddy who shares the same goals as you? The examples are endless.

Strengthening your resolve and knowing yourself are both prerequisites to goal setting. Your mind is ready and you can use your strengths and weaknesses to set a plan that works for you.

## Hack 3: Set Yourself Goals and Keep These in Sight

Wouldn't it be nice if everyone could lose 30 pounds in just 30 days? It's not always possible. Individuals have different motivations for losing weight that can cause them to lose focus on their diet or hit a plateau that is never surpassed. Since no two people are exactly alike, not even twins, you have to set goals that are achievable for you and keep these goals in sight.

Is it possible for you to exercise three times a week in the gym, swimming, or a different form of exercise? Does your lifestyle allow you to cook all your meals or are you always on the move going from one destination to another for work, children, and your spouse?

You need to keep your priorities in view when setting goals. If at all possible, consider changing a few of those priorities to give losing weight more precedence. One of the major stumbling blocks for people losing weight is to set their goals (weight loss) below other activities or needs. Think of a person who owns their own business. This person needs to make certain their company is making money, they are putting food on their table and able to keep shelter over their heads. Going on vacation may be a goal, but it is so low it never happens because food and shelter are more important.

You are going to have priorities that come before losing weight; however, you also have other activities and desires that can be shuffled lower on the scale of importance. If your children have an activity every night of the school week, plus activities on the weekends, you have an area to scale back. You might change the amount of extracurricular activities; therefore, lowering how much time is needed to drive them around. The other option is using all the time your children are conducting those activities to get in exercise.

For the hour they are at an activity, you can go to a gym, go swimming, or perform exercises at home. You can also take some of that time to cook proper meals. These are just a few of the things you want to think about when setting goals. How can you make your weight loss goals fit into your life?

If you have tried losing weight before and been unsuccessful what happened? Did you plateau, fall off the diet, or give up? What caused you to miss the mark on those occasions? Sometimes looking at your failures can help you understand how to create achievable goals this time.

It is not unreasonable for you to set a weight loss goal of 2 pounds a week, but for most people trying to lose a pound a day is not possible. Metabolism, health, and body type all determine the limitations you have in losing weight over time.

# Part Two: You CAN Teach an Old Dog New Tricks

Human nature is to be lazy and stay in a cycle of ease—it takes a lot of mental effort for the brain to learn a new process and eventually make them a habit. However, you can teach yourself new habits in order to help you lose weight and stick to your new exercise and diet regime.

## Hack 4: Hack the Habit Cycle

YOU are the SUM of all your habits. What you are, what you achieve and your success is based on your behaviors and routines. David Eagleman, author of Incognito, writes "Brains are in the business of gathering information and steering behavior appropriately. It doesn't matter whether consciousness is involved in the decision making. And most of the time, it's not." This means if we are going to make any tangible change, we must understand the habit cycle and how we can use it to our advantage.

The brain is a very powerful, if not fully understood organ that drives productivity with the idea of being more efficient. Many tasks and behaviors become habits ensuring we do not have to think with our consciousness, yet still perform. It is great that our brains can function on habits, however, it also leads to bad habits, which are difficult to break. It also makes it hard to gain new habits.

Learning a new task is about processing information. As soon as the brain has learned this task, it becomes an automatic activity, thereby reducing the mental activity or conscious thought required to perform the task. Think back to when you first learnt to tie a tie for example. It seemed pretty hard when you were learning it and you were conscious of every movement and your coordination. But as you learnt it and mastered the technique, it became second nature.

A habit is usually preceded by a trigger – something that initiates the process and ends with a reward. For example, if you think of brushing your teeth. It is preceded by waking up (trigger) and ends with that fresh feeling in your mouth (reward). Try brushing your teeth without toothpaste – I can guarantee that you (your mind) will miss that fresh feeling in your mouth.

Breaking the cycle is NOT about breaking the loop: Trigger -> Action -> Reward. Instead, you need to find a reward that is just as appealing as the bad habit reward. Perhaps you like to eat dessert after each meal. You work hard all day and you feel you deserve a little reward for what has occurred throughout that day. But dessert most likely won't fit your plan, so what can you replace it with something else. Perhaps you enjoy sunsets? You might be a person who can feel great after running, yoga, or swimming? Another person might enjoy 30 minutes to themselves instead of being with their kids and spouse, friends, or other family.

Breaking the habit cycle begins with finding a new reward, but there is more to it than that. Sometimes the reward is not enough to replace the bad habit. Other times you just need plenty of repetition until your brain has accepted the reward as one you crave (brushing your teeth). Only when a reward turns into a craving will your brain automatically choose the healthier routine.

Sadly, backsliding can still occur, even when you start to crave the new reward. Extreme stress can cause us to stick with habits that make us feel even better than the replacement. It means the bad habit can come back two months, six months, or a year after we crave a new reward due to stress.

Charles Duhigg in his book, "The Power of Habit" writes it is only with the support of a group that we can finally stop backsliding and stick to the changes being made. The help of individuals who will not enable our bad habits, but helps us remain on the changed path is necessary. In times where people are stressed and near reverting to their old habits, a helpful hand can stop the slide.

Duhigg cites Alcoholics Anonymous as an example. Many people stop drinking, forming a new, better habit, but can backslide during stressful times or when the reward is seemingly too great to pass up. It is in those times that having a sponsor to call during a weak moment can help you stay on the new routine.

There must be accountability when implementing new habits. There also has to be the belief that you can do it because you are strong and capable of change.

## Hack 5: Start Small

Begin with a small step. Rome was not built in a day. It took decades for the Roman Empire to expand, conquer, and rise to the power it once was. There were many failures, as well as successes. You have to face losing weight with the same mindset. There will be failures, but as long as you have your mind on your goals, work on changing your habit cycles, and have people around you who can help when you need it, you can succeed.

Starting small requires you to cut out certain things. Perhaps it is sugar or fat. You might leave the morning donut in the store instead of having it or maybe take the stairs instead of the elevator. It sounds plausible to start small, but even here you can have challenges.

Consider coffee and soda. Soda is extremely high in sugar, and many sodas are high in caffeine. Caffeine in and of itself is not an appropriate beverage. Cutting out caffeine can be extremely difficult not just because of the cravings, but the body's response to its loss. Headaches and irritability occur when less caffeine is ingested. Yet, you can start small and wean yourself off of the sugary coffee and sodas you drink.

Start by reducing the amount you take in each day. If you drink three cans of soda, make it two. If you drink lattes, mochas and fraps change to black coffee with a little milk or cream. Slowly add decaf to your cup of regular coffee, until you are drinking all decaf. These are just a few suggestions to help you change your habits. You are still getting what your body desires, but in the process of giving yourself a newer, healthier reward, you are also cutting down on caffeine that can cause headaches and irritability. It's sort of similar to a smoker giving up cigarettes and suffering from nicotine withdrawal symptoms.

You want to work on each of your bad habits one at a time and come up with an appropriate reward for each. Replacing dessert with a fruit cup still provides the carbohydrates and sugar taste, albeit differently, but it is a small step in eliminating sugary desserts that are not healthy for you.

If you are not used to exercising or do not like exercising, then you will have to break the cycle you are in by starting small and providing a reward that is still healthy. For example, start exercising just 10 minutes a day. After you exercise, have a treat. The treat can be a smoothie, 10 minutes to relax, 10 minutes of reading a book, or something else you find rewarding that is healthy for you. Once you get into the cycle of exercising and providing a reward, you will form a new habit.

Keeping the habit is difficult, more so if you do not like to exercise in gyms or fitness centers. If possible, try exercising outside with walks in the park, hiking, or other activities you enjoy. Even miniature golfing can be exercise. You are walking, bending, and moving when you golf. Any movement can help; especially, if you are used to being sedentary. The trick is to start small and reward yourself with healthy benefits.

## Hack 6: Hack your Brain to use Cravings to your Advantage

Now that you know the science behind the habit cycle, you can start to use new cravings to retain your healthy habits. When your body craves something that is not good for you, you tend to dwell on it. You imagine munching on a bag of your favorite chips, candy, or other snacks.

Go ahead and imagine your favorite snack right now. How do you feel? Are you hoping you have that snack in your kitchen or are you already reaching for it? With cravings a single mention of the word can trigger your desire to have that item. It doesn't seem fair that your brain can have that much power over you, but it does.

You can take advantage of these cravings to correct your brain. There are two experts in the field who study cravings and rewiring your brain that can help us understand, according to Thorin Klosowski. Wilhelm Hofmann and Dr. Kelly McGonigal have thoroughly studied willpower and the ability to correct your brain.

Cravings are generated from the reward part of the habit cycle. A craving is something that the brain brings into a more conscious level, so we will act on it. There is a feeling of "longing." Your mind can start picturing a bag of chips, how rewarding it is to eat them, how they taste and even feel on our tongues. Suddenly the entire bag can be eaten.

It is both a physical and psychological need. Physical cravings are less apparent than psychological ones. The body typically has cravings for things it has gotten used to, such as alcohol, food, and other things. The physical aspect is like an addiction, but we don't consider it one unless we relate it to drugs or alcohol. Yet, the cravings can be every bit as addictive, particularly when you cannot control the amount of reward you "must have." Dr. McGonigal believes cravings began with survival and reproduction. The brain and body crave what it requires to survive. However, over time we started to let these "cravings into the rest of our lives." It has led us to consume things we do not need for survival.

The psychology of cravings is a little different. The body's reward system identifies a certain thing it wants. The brain then releases dopamine. Dopamine is a chemical associated with happiness or pleasure. Your desire for gratification blocks any goal you have against the craving you have. Your prefrontal cortex is telling you not to eat what you crave; all the while the good feelings want you to have a short-term fulfilment.

Your brain will release stress hormones due to the debate. It tells you the discomfort you feel can only be corrected if you start appeasing that craving. The unfortunate part is that our brains can teach us that almost anything is a reward. It can turn a behavior into a compulsion.

Knowing how cravings work is just the beginning of solving the issue. Get something you crave—one you know that provides a false reward. It can be cookies, chips, cake, or anything. Eat as much as you can. This is a test of your emotions. At first you are happy. Next you start to crave the food more. The taste becomes more enhanced. Once you reach the point of eating too much of that food your body tells you that you still want more. Despite not being satisfied your body is telling you to eat more of that food. It is also telling you that you are full or feeling nauseous because you ate too much.

The goal of this exercise is to help rewire your brain. You need to focus on the bad feelings you have after eating that food. The consequence is feeling horrible after eating it. If you focus your mind on those feelings, you can trick your body into forgetting about the rewarding feeling.

The key is to provide instant gratification through a proper reward, allowing you to stick to your long term goals. Here are some suggestions:

1. Form motivations that compete with cravings. Help your body recognize a motivation versus a craving. Remember, you created goals? The constant reminder of your goals helps you switch your brain from automatic cravings and seeking rewards to the long term goals. It helps you modify your brain into thinking cravings are the negative effect.


2. If necessary, repeat the test with the food you ate too much of. You can test other foods. You need to remind your body of how it felt after you ate the food, after you were full and feeling unwell. Dwell on those feelings with the foods that are not healthy for you. Let your mind remember that the instant reward led to a horrible feeling.


3. The next step is to handle the trigger when it is present. You need to avoid succumbing to the trigger. You can do this by changing or altering your environment. You might have a something you do not like. For example, you might find you are more susceptible to eating junk food at the office because of the stress you feel with paperwork. You can move from your office to a coffee shop, eat a healthy snack and retrain your brain. If you do not like exercising, but love shopping, go window shopping or shopping.


You are getting exercise and a reward. Dopamine will eventually stop being released, but you have had plenty of time to create a new, healthier habit. If you cannot move offices, adding in new pictures, furniture, or items from home that make you happy can help. You can change your home too by placing running shoes at the door, putting healthy food where you kept the junk, and basically triggering your brain with the healthier option.

Changing your brain to use cravings to your advantage is about adapting all areas of your life. For example, stress due to overspending can lead to eating improperly. You can use these steps to stop overspending, save money instead, and then correct your eating habits. Sometimes you have to find the cause of the weight gain before you can lose the weight.

## Hack 7: Social Motivation

Social motivation is a highly effective form of motivation which can help you with your goals. Being with a group of people who are just as willing to lose weight helps remind you of your goals. Someone can say "are you really going to eat that?" to help remind you that your choice in that moment can have a negative effect on your long term goal.

Sometimes, being in a group of like-minded individuals helps. At other times you may not need the group. You could post pictures on social media as a motivator.

Start with a picture of how you look now. For most that are overweight they are not too happy to see their reflection in the camera. It can cause embarrassment to post such an image. But this is motivation. If you do not like how you look and how others will see you, then posting an image of yourself before the weight loss is a public reminder.

It is also a way for you to make a pledge. You can pledge to lose x amount of pounds this month. It is public. It is embarrassing or uncomfortable if you do not reach that goal. It can be a good motivator to keep you going, it also gives your friends a way to say "way to go," "keep up the good work," "how's it going with your goal?" and many other things to help keep you motivated.

When you reach the goal, you will post a new picture. This new picture is the reward. It shows you lost x amount of pounds. You reached the goal. Now it is time for a new goal. You can continue on that cycle until you have reached the main goal—whatever amount of weight you wanted to lose when you began.

Social media also gives you a way to connect with others who are struggling just as much or perhaps more than you are. Some of your friends may be just as embarrassed about their weight gain, but are hiding it. You can help show them it is not that scary and there is potential for making those goals. It is another reward that you gain during your process of weight loss—the reward of helping others.

Social media and group motivation can be a helpful element to your diet and overall weight loss. However, you also need to choose your social interactions carefully.

Not everyone is equal in the amount of help they can provide. Depending on the wrong person to help you when you need to stick to your weight loss goals may create failures. You may feel down or more stressed.

You need to create a team that will help you in your goals by being supportive and happy for you, without judging or enabling you. The person that says "Oh, it's just a little piece of pie" is not helping.  The trigger is present and your craving is there, it just needs a nudge.

Luckily, there are plenty of social options to help you hack your brain the right way. Social diet programs are a great way to get the help from fellow weight loss gurus, without feeling alone in the entire process. But always keep one thing in mind—your motivation and strengths are what will ultimately carry you through to your goal. Believing in yourself and making it happen is because of your inner strength.

# Part 3: Failure is an Option

"Failure is not an option" is a negative phrase that is too often used. Throughout life we are taught that failure, any failure is not acceptable. If "you fail, you are a loser." These horrible negative statements are wrong. **Failure is an option**. If you need to, look at history. Do you think Warren Buffet became the businessman he is today without failures? Do you think Edison was successful in every invention he created? The examples are numerous

## Hack 8: Allow yourself to Fail

Allow yourself to fail; you are only a human being. Mistakes and missed goals occur. You are going to feel bad when it happens. You may feel like it is pointless to try and lose weight. Everyone on a diet and weight loss program has felt these feelings. It is how you react that will make the difference. You might stop the diet that you thought would be the one successful option. You might have misinterpreted what the diet was asking of you. There are many reasons failure can result, but you are only human. Your path to losing weight and becoming healthier will not end as long as you are living and determined.

The key is to remember your training with setting up achievable goals and training your brain to use habits and cravings to your advantage. You have learned the secrets to overwriting the wrongs in your brain. You have the willpower to succeed no matter what happens.

There are certain things you need to remember when it comes to dieting. Your body will lose weight wonderfully for a short time. It will be energized with the proper health foods and new exercise, but you will reach a plateau. Every person reaches a point where they cannot seem to lose any more weight. It happens to celebrities all the time. Some celebrities lose the weight and gain it right back. No one is immune to the human condition.

How you deal with the failure when it happens, is what matters. Yes, this diet didn't get you to your goal, maybe you hit a plateau? You can "trick" your body to lose more weight. It may be as simple as changing the type of exercises you are doing. You might increase your calories to help give your metabolism a boost.

Concentrate on the positive feelings, on the rewards you have gotten from the diet, and let go of the negative consequences. If necessary, you can think of the negative as a motivator. For some failure is a very strong motivator to succeed the next time. It will depend on your personality; whether the positive or the negative is a greater motivator to keep you working on losing the weight.

## Hack 9: Give yourself a Break

Give yourself a break from time to time. You can decide when this is, every 2 weeks, every 2 months or every time you have made a mistake and failed on your diet. It doesn't mean to stop working towards new habit cycles, with better cravings and a healthier outlook. When you give yourself a break, you are stepping back, realizing your limitations, mistakes, and looking for the answer on how to correct what has led to failures (if any).

Having a break also gives you time to enjoy some of the more frivolous aspects of life! This doesn't mean you are a failure at sticking to your goals, it allows you to realize and remember that you only have one life.

The problems occur when people have this mindset for extended periods of time. Life is all about balance!

Remember, you are only human. There are limitations to what you can do, even with your own body. It is always a good idea to get a complete physical and have an entire blood panel run before starting any weight loss regime. However, if you have not done that and experienced a weight loss/diet failure before—do it now. You never know what health problem could be forcing a plateau or worse—no weight loss at all.

## Hack 10: Starvation is the Enemy

Mistakes can be made during any diet and weight loss program. For some individuals' mistakes are derived from fad diets that promise magical results in a short time. For others, it can be forgetting that there is power in numbers. Starvation is one of the biggest mistakes dieters make in trying to lose weight quickly. You need to eat and give your body the appropriate nutrients.

The science behind how your body and mind works can be broken into the two concepts mentioned in previous chapters: survival and reproduction. When it comes right down to it, any human is programmed for survival and reproduction. You cannot ignore this simple fact.

Your body will do anything it can to survive, including preventing weight loss. When you starve yourself, you will see some weight loss. Eventually, after a couple of weeks or a month, your body will stop losing weight and start storing it with anything you do take in. You won't be burning calories during exercise, except for the minimal amount it takes to keep you functioning.

Other parts of your body will cease to function. Your mind will slow down; shutting down some automatic processes it does not require to keep your body moving.

With enough starvation, important organs can start to shut down and death can occur. Long before this, most people cave. They go back to the foods they craved before and start binging. The mind starts to overrule the weight loss desire to the point that the opposite occurs.

Your diet and exercise regime should never include starvation. Detox diets, where you are able to drink only clear liquids or eat clear liquids will certainly cause weight loss in the first few weeks. However, after three days you must start eating properly again if you want to continue to lose weight. It is the reason most detox diets provide a short jumpstart before getting into well planned, well balanced meals.

According to expert nutritionists around the world, your body needs at least 1,000 calories a day to function properly and still allow for weight loss. Anything less than 1,000 calories will immediately put your body into survival mode and you will not see the weight disappear.

Starving does not have to be under 1,000 calories. You cannot suddenly go from eating 2k or 3k calories in a day to 1k. You will feel hungry. Your brain will tell you that you are hungry. The cravings for all things bad will appear and you will find you are not satisfied.

Make certain you are eating a proper, balanced diet each day.

## A Final Note

This book was an attempt at helping millions of other reach their goals. I hope that you have found these hacks useful. Remember, your mind is your greatest treasure, cultivate it and reap the benefits not just in respects to weight loss, but every aspect in your life.

I would love to hear about your progress with your goals and how this guide has helped you.

If you enjoyed this book and believe it provided value to you, I would love it if you could give it a review: this will help me reach so many more people!

Made in the USA
Las Vegas, NV
29 December 2024

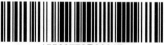